PREVENTING LEAD EXPOSURE IN YOUNG CHILDREN:
A Housing-Based Approach to Primary Prevention of Lead Poisoning

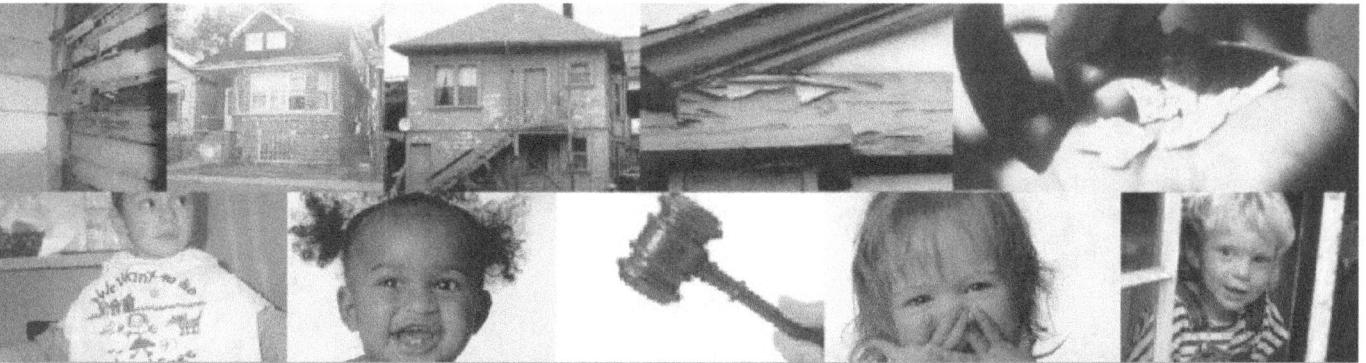

RECOMMENDATIONS FROM THE ADVISORY COMMITTEE ON
CHILDHOOD LEAD POISONING PREVENTION

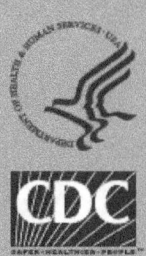

Preventing Lead Exposure in Young Children:

Preventing Lead Exposure in Young Children:
A Housing-Based Approach to Primary Prevention of Lead Poisoning

RECOMMENDATIONS FROM THE ADVISORY COMMITTEE ON
CHILDHOOD LEAD POISONING PREVENTION

Centers for Disease Control and Prevention
Julie L. Gerberding, MD, MPH, Director

National Center for Environmental Health
Henry Falk, MD, MPH, Director

Division of Emergency and Environmental Health Services
Jim Rabb, Acting Director

Lead Poisoning Prevention Branch
Mary Jean Brown, ScD, RN, Chief

**U.S. Department of Health
and Human Services, Public Health Service**

October 2004

Suggested reference: Centers for Disease Control and Prevention. Preventing Lead Exposure in Young Children: A Housing-Based Approach to Primary Prevention of Lead Poisoning. Atlanta: CDC;2004.

Contents

Preventing Lead Exposure in Young Children:

Acknowledgements

The Advisory Committee on Childhood Lead Poisoning Prevention acknowledges the contributions of the late Ellis Goldman, who assisted with manuscript development and editing. Ellis was a colleague and true friend whose dedication to the primary prevention of childhood lead poisoning continues to inspire us all.

We thank the members of the Primary Prevention Work Group for their hard work and dedication in the initial conception, development, writing and revision of this manuscript. We acknowledge the sterling leadership of Amy Murphy (first Work Group chairperson) in guiding the process, and the efforts of Work Group members Richard Bunner, Cushing Dolbeare, Anne M. Guthrie, David Jacobs, Susan Klitzman, Bruce P. Lanphear, Ronald Morony, Pamela Meyer and Tim Morta.

We also acknowledge the valuable and extensive contributions of CDC staff members including Crystal Gresham, Janet Henry, Nikki Kilpatrick, Tim Morta, Philip Jacobs, Marcia Brooks, Linda Anderson and Mary Jean Brown.

Rachel Wilson provided editorial support.

Special thanks should go to the public health professionals who reviewed the document and provided helpful and practical suggestions for improvement: Valerie Charlton (California), John Domzalski (Philadelphia), Richard Leiker (Oregon), Andrea Michael (Minnesota), Ed Norman (North Carolina), David Schor (Ohio), and Richard Tobin (Philadelphia).

Pat McLaine,
Chairperson, Primary Prevention Work Group

Carla Campbell,
Chairperson, Advisory Committee on Childhood Lead Poisoning Prevention

Executive Summary

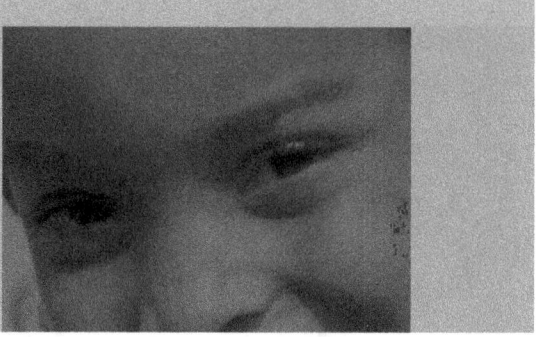

This document presents recommendations from the Centers for Disease Control and Prevention's (CDC) Advisory Committee on Childhood Lead Poisoning Prevention (ACCLPP) for a housing-based approach to primary prevention of childhood lead poisoning to accelerate progress toward achieving the *Healthy People 2010* objective of eliminating elevated blood lead levels (BLLs), defined as at or above 10 micrograms per deciliter (≥ 10 µg/dL), in children.[1] Childhood lead exposure and its resultant clinical manifestations ranging from elevated BLLs to frank lead poisoning remain a major public health problem among young children in the United States. Lead adversely affects children's cognitive and behavioral development, which is strongly related to their future productivity and expected earnings. Dramatic reductions in BLLs of U.S. children during 1970 - 1990 were attributed to population-based primary prevention policies (such as the banning of lead in gasoline) in conjunction with improved lead screening and identification of children with elevated BLLs. Estimates based on 1999 - 2000 nationally representative data suggest that about 2.2% of children aged 1 - 5 years (about 434,000 children) have elevated BLLs.[2] Research suggests that these elevated BLLs result primarily from exposure to lead in nonintact paint, interior settled dust, and exterior soil and dust in and around older deteriorating housing. Renovation in older housing also creates substantial lead hazards unless dust is contained and the areas are thoroughly cleaned. Although many sources of lead exposure exist for children, the recommendations in this report focus on preventing childhood exposure to lead-based paint hazards in and around housing.

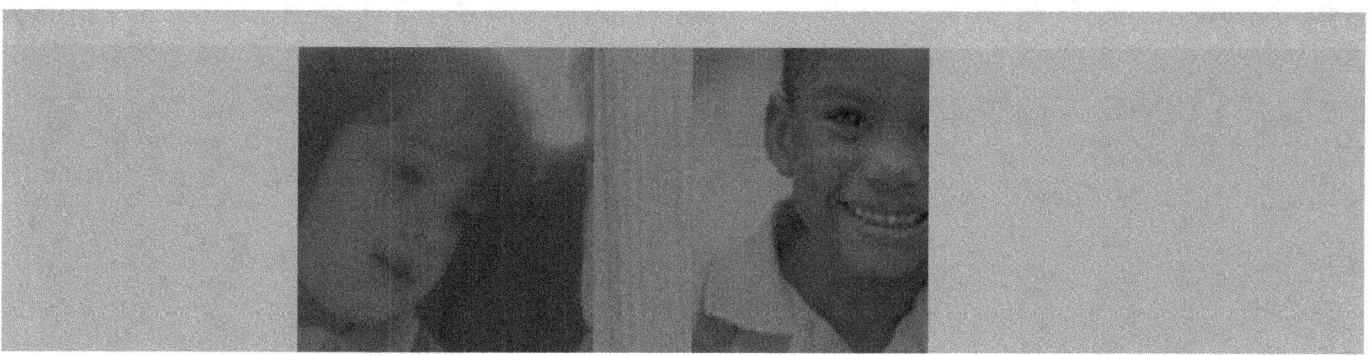

ACCLPP fully supports the concept of local and state decision-making to determine the most appropriate blood lead screening approach based on local conditions and data, which was the centerpiece of the revised 1997 guidelines. Efforts to ensure that the health care system incorporates these guidelines are extremely important. Most childhood lead poisoning prevention programs focus on identification and management of individual cases of elevated BLLs (i.e., secondary prevention). Follow-up care for such children consists of education focused on lead hazards, behavior changes associated with lead exposure, medical and developmental follow-up, nutritional recommendations, and environmental interventions.[3] Environmental interventions to control identified lead hazards and halt further exposure may not be carried out because of lack of resources and/or statutory authority. Evidence suggests that the benefits of secondary prevention are limited. However, identification and provision of services to children with elevated BLLs remain important components of a comprehensive lead poisoning prevention program. To ensure successful elimination of elevated BLLs in children, programs must not rely solely on screening and secondary prevention but also focus on preventing lead exposure through the implementation of housing-based primary prevention.

The actions recommended in this report can be performed by an array of entities, including health departments and other public agencies, community-based agencies, and the private sector. Health departments must provide leadership to increase knowledge about lead safety and to encourage broad action to make housing lead-safe (i.e., a condition in which lead-based paint hazards have been eliminated or controlled by trained or certified contractors). To accomplish these goals, health departments must assume a leadership role in fostering collaboration among housing agencies, elected officials, and other stakeholders. Recent developments in technology and national housing policy can help to correct unsafe housing, the primary vector of lead exposure. This document provides a rationale for emphasizing primary prevention and an outline of a comprehensive program based on eight core elements (See "Eight Elements of a Comprehensive Program for Primary Prevention of Childhood Lead Poisoning" on page 11).

Specific examples of recommended program elements in use are documented through a CDC-funded project titled, *Building Blocks for Primary Prevention: Protecting Children from Lead-Based Paint Hazards*, that was initiated in October 2002. Because even the most intense primary prevention efforts to increase the supply of lead-safe housing will take years, childhood lead poisoning prevention programs (CLPPPs) should continue to augment their systemic housing-based primary prevention changes with fast-track initiatives to identify high-risk families who could benefit from immediate assessment and risk-reduction services to prevent further childhood lead exposure. With the shift towards primary prevention, program evaluation efforts should be a research priority so that future commitments of resources can focus on cost-effectively achieving program and national goals to reduce childhood lead exposure.

...program evaluation efforts should be a research priority...

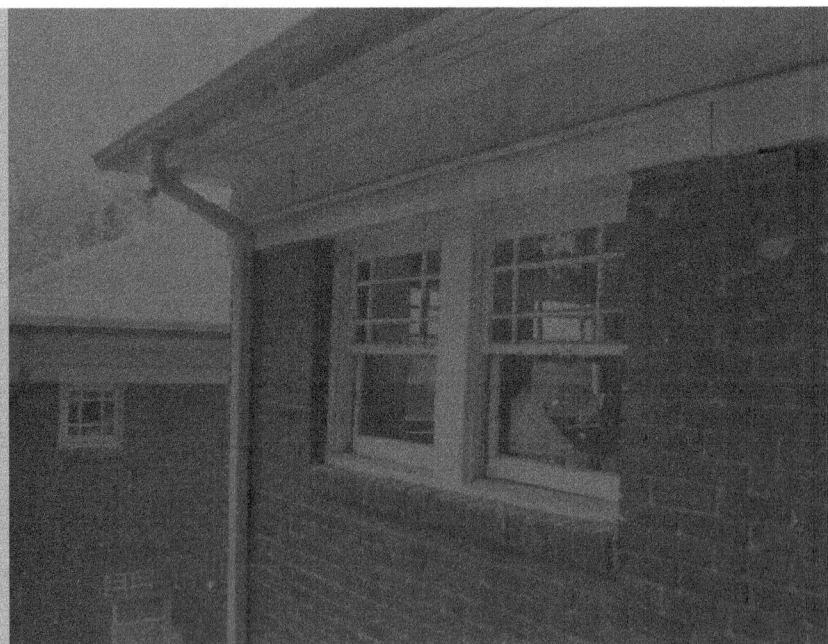

Eight Elements of a Comprehensive Program for Primary Prevention of Childhood Lead Poisoning

1. Identify high-risk areas, populations, and activities associated with housing-based lead exposure.

2. Use local data and expertise to expand resources and motivate action for primary prevention.

3. Develop strategies and ensure services for creating lead-safe housing.

4. Develop and codify specifications for lead-safe housing treatments.

5. Strengthen regulatory infrastructure necessary to create lead-safe housing.

6. Engage in collaborative plans and programs with housing and other appropriate agencies.

7. Evaluate and redesign existing **CLPPP** elements to achieve primary prevention goals while ensuring adequate secondary interventions.

8. Evaluate primary prevention progress and identify research opportunities.

Members of the Advisory Committee on Childhood Lead Poisoning Prevention

CHAIR

Carla Campbell, MD, MS
The Children's Hospital of Philadelphia
Philadelphia, Pennsylvania

EXECUTIVE SECRETARY

Mary Jean Brown, ScD, RN
Chief, Lead Poisoning Prevention Branch
National Center for Environmental Health
Centers for Disease Control and Prevention
Atlanta, Georgia

MEMBERS

William Banner, Jr., MD, PhD
The Children's Hospital at Saint Francis
Tulsa, Oklahoma

Helen J. Binns, MD, MPH
Children's Memorial Hospital
Chicago, Illinois

Cushing N. Dolbeare *
Housing and Policy Consultant
Mitchellville, Maryland

Anne M. Guthrie, MPH *
Alliance for Healthy Homes
Washington, D.C.

Walter S. Handy, Jr., PhD
Cincinnati Health Department
Cincinnati, Ohio

Birt Harvey, MD *
Pediatrician
Palo Alto, California

Ing Kang Ho, PhD
University of Mississippi Medical Center
Jackson, Mississippi

Richard E. Hoffman, MD, MPH
Physician
Denver, Colorado

Jessica Leighton, PhD, MPH
New York City Department of Health & Mental Hygiene
New York, New York

Tracey V. Lynn, DVM, MS
Alaska Department of Health and Social Services
Anchorage, Alaska

Sergio Piomelli, MD
Columbia Presbyterian Medical Center
New York, New York

Michael W. Shannon, MD, MPH †
Children's Hospital
Boston, Massachusetts

Catherine M. Slota-Varma, MD
Pediatrician
Milwaukee, Wisconsin

Kevin U. Stephens, Sr., MD, JD
New Orleans Department of Health
New Orleans, LA

Kimberly M. Thompson, ScD
Harvard School of Public Health
Boston, Massachusetts

* ACCLPP member until June 2003
† ACCLPP member until April 2003

EX-OFFICIO MEMBERS

Agency for Toxic Substance and Disease Registry
Olivia Harris, MA

Centers for Disease Control and Prevention
Robert J. Roscoe, MS

Centers for Medicare and Medicaid Services
Jerry Zelinger, MD

Food and Drug Administration
Michael P. Bolger, PhD

Health Resources & Services Administration
Byron P. Bailey, MPH

National Institute for Environmental Health Sciences
Walter Rogan, MD

U.S. Agency for International Development
John Borrazzo, PhD

U.S. Consumer Product Safety Commission
Lori Saltzman

U.S. Department of Housing and
Urban Development
David Jacobs, PhD, CIH

U.S. Environmental Protection Agency
Ronald J. Morony, PE

LIAISON REPRESENTATIVES

American Academy of Pediatrics
J. Routt Reigart, II, MD

American Association of Poison Control Centers
George C. Rodgers, Jr., MD, PhD

American Industrial Hygiene Association
Steve M. Hays, CIH, PE

American Public Health Association
Patricia Nolan, MD, MPH

Association of Public Health Laboratories
Henry Bradford, Jr., PhD

Association of State and Territorial
Health Officials
Karen Pearson

Council of State and Territorial Epidemiologists
Ezatollah Keyvan-Larijani, MD, DrPH

National Center for Healthy Housing
Pat McLaine, RN, MPH

Primary Prevention Work Group

Pat McLaine, RN, MPH, Chairperson
National Center for Healthy Housing
Columbia, Maryland

Amy Murphy, MPH Chairperson
(November 2001 - March 2003)
City of Milwaukee Health Department
Milwaukee, Wisconsin

Richard Bunner, MPH
Ohio Department of Health
Columbus, Ohio

Carla Campbell, MD, MS
The Children's Hospital of Philadelphia
Philadelphia, Pennsylvania

Cushing Dolbeare
Housing Policy Consultant
Mitchellville, Maryland

Anne M. Guthrie, MPH
Alliance for Healthy Homes
Washington, D.C.

David Jacobs, PhD, CIH
U.S. Department of Housing and
Urban Development
Washington, D.C.

Susan Klitzman, DrPH
Hunter College
New York, New York

Bruce P. Lanphear, MD, MPH
Children's Hospital Medical Center
Cincinnati, Ohio

Pamela Meyer, PhD
Centers for Disease Control and Prevention
Atlanta, Georgia

Ronald Morony, PE
U.S. Environmental Protection Agency
Washington, D.C.

Tim Morta
Centers for Disease Control and Prevention
Atlanta, Georgia

Glossary

Abatement-A measure or set of measures designed to permanently eliminate lead-based paint hazards and/or lead-based paint. (Source: HUD and EPA)

At-risk populations-Children aged <6 years (especially those aged 0 - 3 years) and pregnant women who occupy homes constructed before 1978, and Medicaid-enrolled and Medicaid-eligible children. (This definition will be further refined on the basis of local conditions and data.)

Case management-The follow-up care of a child with an elevated blood lead level. Case management includes a) client identification and outreach; b) individual assessment and diagnosis; c) service planning and resource identification; d) linkage of clients to needed services; e) service implementation and coordination; f) monitoring of service delivery; g) advocacy; and h) evaluation. (CDC)

Clearance standards-Maximum allowable lead dust* levels on surfaces (e.g., floors, windowsills, and window wells) after a residence has undergone lead hazard control work. (CDC)

Clearance examination-Visual examination and collection of lead dust samples by an inspector or risk assessor and analysis by an accredited laboratory upon completion of an abatement project, interim control intervention, or maintenance job that disturbs lead-based paint (or paint suspected of being lead-based) above the minimus levels. HUD and EPA have established maximum allowable lead dust levels on surfaces (e.g., floors, window sills, and window troughs). (HUD)

Consolidated Plan-A plan required and approved by HUD for state and local grantees that receive federal housing and/or community development block grants that set forth the jurisdiction's statement of the housing problems, its 5-year plan to address the identified problems, and a 1-year action plan.

Distressed housing- Residential property in poor physical condition or likely to fall into such condition because of deferred maintenance, which typically has multiple structural problems, code violations, and lead hazards.Distressed housing is typically older, occupied by very low income households or abandoned, and requires major investment of resources to correct structural deficiencies, repair building systems, and control health and safety problems.

Elevated blood lead level-Blood lead level ≥ 10 $\mu g/dL$. (CDC)

Essential maintenance practices-Approved maintenance practices and procedures designed to control deteriorating paint and/or lead dust that are undertaken regularly to ensure a home is maintained in a lead-safe condition. These practices involve dust and paint chip containment using "wet" procedures and specialized cleanup.

Interim controls-A set of measures designed to temporarily reduce human exposure to lead-based paint hazards. (HUD)

Lead hazard-Accessible paint, dust, soil, water, or other source or pathway that contains lead or lead compounds that can contribute to or cause elevated BLLs. (CDC)

Lead hazard control-Activities, including interim measures and permanent abatement, to control and eliminate lead hazards. (EPA)

Lead hazard screen-A limited environmental screening activity focused on visual assessment, which may include paint, dust and soil sampling and is usually performed in housing units less likely to contain lead-based paint hazards or as a preliminary step in the lead hazard assessment process.*

Lead-based paint-Paint or other surface coating that contains lead equal to or exceeding 1.0 milligram per square centimeter or 0.5% by weight or 5,000 parts per million by weight. (HUD and EPA)

Lead risk assessment-An onsite investigation of a residential dwelling to discover any lead-based paint hazards and description of options to eliminate them, which includes lead dust and soil sampling. (HUD and EPA)

Lead-safe-Housing with no lead paint hazards as determined by a lead risk assessment or by dust sampling at the conclusion of lead hazard control activities. If lead-based paint remains in the housing unit, its condition and any hazard control systems must be monitored to prevent new lead hazards.

Lead-safe maintenance-See Essential maintenance practices

Lead-safe work practices-Low-technology practices for general renovation, repainting, and maintenance projects that control, contain, and clean up lead dust and deteriorated lead-based paint in a manner that protects both the workers and the occupants of the unit being treated.

Lien-A legal instrument used by a court to impose a requirement upon a property owner for the satisfaction of some debt or duty.

---

* Some states have calibrated lead safety measures to a property's risk, establishing tiered requirements for different circumstances, including 2002 laws enacted in Rhode Island and Maryland.

Paint inspection-A surface-by-surface investigation to determine the presence of lead-based paint (may include dust and soil sampling) and a report of the results. (HUD and EPA)

Primary prevention-Interventions undertaken to reduce or eliminate exposures or risk factors before the onset of detectable disease. This includes measures to a) prevent the dispersal of lead in the environment through regulations or other measures that prevent harmful uses of lead and b) remove lead from the environment before children are exposed. (CDC)

Receivership-A condition in which a person or entity is appointed to receive and hold in trust a property under litigation.

Rehabilitation-Actions taken in which a building is physically modified, either to improve the condition of the structure or to change its use.

Remediation-Physical intervention in a building to control and/or eliminate identified deficiencies or hazards and render the building safe.

Renovation-Construction and/or home or building improvement measures (e.g., window replacement, weatherization, remodeling, and repairing). (HUD)

Satisfactory compliance-The conduct of both visual and laboratory (i.e., dust) tests by certified personnel and an accredited laboratory to ensure that the lead hazard control work completed in a home has rendered the unit lead-safe (commonly known as "clearance" within the context of lead hazard control) and has met applicable standards for work and lead safety.

Secondary prevention-Response to a problem after it has been detected. This involves identifying children with elevated BLLs and eliminating or reducing their lead exposure. (CDC)

Introduction

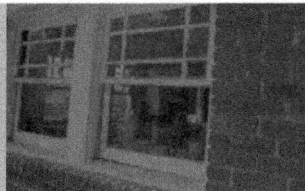

This document presents recommendations developed by the Centers for Disease Control and Prevention's (CDC) Advisory Committee on Childhood Lead Poisoning Prevention (ACCLPP) through its Primary Prevention Work Group. This document emphasizes primary prevention of childhood lead poisoning to accelerate progress toward achieving the *Healthy People 2010* Objective 8-11: the elimination of elevated blood lead levels (BLLs) in children.[1] To reach this objective, changes are required at the state and local levels, where childhood lead poisoning prevention programs (CLPPPs) must initiate and collaborate with other groups and agencies in implementing housing-based primary prevention strategies that work at the community level. Therefore, this document is directed primarily toward the state and local health departments responsible for childhood lead poisoning (including those with CLPPPs), local programs funded by the U.S. Department of Housing and Urban Development (HUD), and all other partners in primary prevention.

Dramatic reductions in BLLs of U.S. children during 1970 - 1990 were attributed to population-based environmental policies that banned the use of lead in gasoline, paint, drinking-water conduits, food and beverage containers, and other products that created widespread exposure to lead.[4,5] These primary prevention efforts reflect one of the great public health successes of the 20th century.[6] These lead level reductions were achieved in conjunction with improved lead screening and identification of children with elevated BLLs. Because of the reduction in average BLLs in children from an estimated 15 µg/dL in 1976 - 1980[7] to approximately 2 µg/dL in 1999,[2] the cohort of children who reach age 2 each year may reap an estimated annual benefit as high as $110 - $319 billion from the prevented losses of future earning potential alone due to improved workforce participation and higher salaries.[8]

Despite these gains in public health, lead exposure continues to affect young children in the United States. The limits of secondary prevention (i.e., implementing measures after a child has an elevated BLL) as a way to eliminate childhood lead poisoning increasingly are being recognized. The estimated average skeletal lead concentrations of contemporary humans is 500- to 1000-fold higher than that of preindustrial humans,[9] and an increasing body of scientific information has identified harmful health effects associated with BLLs lower than were previously considered "safe."[10-13] Disparities by income and race are well-documented.[5-7, 14]

Because children are exposed to lead from a variety of sources and no discernable threshold has been defined for the adverse effects of lead, reducing all environmental sources of lead exposure (including lead from past uses that remains in the environment) is necessary. Residential lead hazards are the primary source of lead intake for U.S. children. However, numerous other sources of lead intake for U.S. children have been identified and vary by location.[3] Examples are the use of ethnic remedies;[15] cosmetics;[16] lead-containing ceramics;[17] vinyl mini-blinds;[18] lead brought from a work-site into the home by a parent;[19,20] and products such as crayons and toys that have been contaminated with lead. However, each of these products probably constitute a significant source of lead intake for only a small number of children. Industrial point sources, smelters, and power plant emissions also can contribute to lead intake in children.[21-24] Reducing lead emissions and the introduction of new lead into the environment may be critical to achieving maximum reductions in lead exposure in areas affected by these sources.[25] Many opportunities remain for eliminating unnecessary lead uses and reducing emissions.

Although many sources of lead can affect certain individuals and communities, the primary source of childhood lead exposure in the United States is lead paint in older, deteriorating housing.[3,14,26] Children are most often exposed to lead in their homes through nonintact paint, interior settled dust, and exterior soil and dust. Renovation of older homes also can cause substantial lead hazards.[27,28] Therefore, the recommendations in this report focus on preventing childhood exposure to lead-based paint hazards in housing.

Most CLPPPs emphasize secondary prevention of lead poisoning (i.e., blood lead screening of children to identify and provide follow-up care for those with elevated BLLs). This approach has limited benefit for most children living in housing that poses an increased risk for lead-associated health effects. However, primary prevention interventions to reduce lead exposures populationwide have succeeded. Primary prevention of lead hazards within the home on an individual or community level requires that lead-based paint hazards in and around homes be identified and controlled before a child is exposed. Many CLPPPs have developed primary prevention activities, but few have made primary prevention their main focus, in major part because of limited resources and authority. In some instances, CLPPPs have emphasized primary prevention measures associated with behavior change (e.g., encouraging families to increase hand washing and wet mopping and achieve recommended levels of iron and calcium intake). However, such educational interventions alone do not significantly reduce exposures and offer little sustainable protection to children whose homes contain peeling paint and lead-dust hazards.[29]

Although the medical and public health communities now possess knowledge of the primary prevention tools needed to do the job, we have yet to marshal the will and resources to accomplish such prevention. Recent trends indicate that the time is right for a concerted effort. In many communities lead caseloads have declined, sometimes in association with a decrease in screening penetration, but more likely paralleling nationwide declines in prevalence of elevated BLLs in children. Many health departments have taken the opportunity afforded by these developments to focus on improving "core" public health functions.[30] For example, many CLPPPs are now able to 1) assess populationwide risk for lead exposure; 2) use data to target interventions and improve service delivery; 3) track lead-related services provided by others (e.g., screening and medical management); and 4) collaborate with partners (e.g., state Medicaid agencies, managed-care organizations, housing agencies, and community-based organizations). As a result, many CLPPPs are poised to assume leadership roles in this shift toward housing-based primary prevention of childhood lead exposure.

The U.S. Department of Health and Human Services (DHHS) and CDC consistently have encouraged state and local health departments and housing agencies to move toward housing-based primary prevention, beginning with the 1991 document titled, *Strategic Plan for the Elimination of Childhood Lead Poisoning*,[31] and the CDC statement, *Preventing Lead Poisoning in Young Children*.[4] Most recently, CDC has begun requiring its grantee health departments and CLPPPs to develop a strategic plan to eliminate childhood lead poisoning and to include primary prevention strategies.[32] ACCLPP recommendations published in the 2002 document, *Managing Elevated Blood Lead Levels in Young Children*,[3] stated, "...primary prevention by the removal of ongoing lead exposure sources should be promoted as the ideal and most effective means of preventing elevated blood lead levels." We present these recommendations to promote this goal and turn it into reality.

Strong support and resource allocation from the federal government will increase the likelihood that state and local initiatives will succeed. Federal agencies have important roles in supporting primary prevention programs by sponsoring research, developing and periodically updating tools and guidance for assessing and monitoring lead safety in housing, insisting on lead-safe practices in all federally supported housing programs, funding lead hazard control and evaluation programs, providing technical assistance, periodically updating regulations, and reviewing federal funding requirements to ensure consistency with primary prevention goals. The ACCLPP recommends that DHHS strengthen its efforts to promote and facilitate primary prevention and maintain a leadership role in collaborating with other federal agencies.

This document is a guideline for accomplishing primary prevention and lowering childhood lead exposure in communities around the nation, which is best achieved through eliminating the three primary exposure pathways (i.e., deteriorated paint, contaminated dust, and contaminated soil) in and around housing. This guideline provides a rationale and an outline of a comprehensive program for developing and implementing a primary prevention strategy (see box), as well as references and resources that may be useful in accomplishing this goal.

L ead adversely affects children's cognitive and behavioral development.[3] Elevated BLLs in children are associated with growth impairment, increased blood pressure, impaired heme synthesis, increases in hearing threshold, and slowed nerve conduction.[33] Lead toxicity economically impacts individuals and society because cognitive ability is strongly correlated with productivity and expected earnings. An increase of 10 µg/dL in a child's BLL may reduce the present value of that child's individual future lifetime earnings by approximately $37,000.[8]

Estimates based on 1999 - 2000 data suggest that about 2.2% of children aged 1 - 5 years (about 434,000 children) have BLLs of $\geq$10 µg/dL.[34] A national survey found that children at highest risk for having an elevated BLL are those living in metropolitan areas and in housing built before 1946, from low-income families, and of African-American and Hispanic origin.[14] Because lead exposure disproportionately affects children in low-income families living in older housing, it represents a significant, preventable contributor to social disparities in health, educational achievement and overall quality of life.

Limits of Secondary Prevention Alone

Intervening after a child's BLL becomes elevated could reduce or prevent further lead exposure but may do little to reverse lead-associated cognitive impairment.[35,36] Most CLPPPs rely on the use of routine blood lead screening to identify children with elevated BLLs. In most areas, follow-up care for children with BLLs 10 - 20 µg/dL consists of education focused on lead hazards, changing behaviors associated with lead exposure, medical and developmental follow-up, nutritional recommendations, and environmental interventions to prevent further exposure.[3] However, children with BLLs $\geq$15 µg/dL generally receive more intensive follow-up services as BLLs increase. Environmental interventions to control identified lead hazards and halt further exposure are sometimes not carried out. For children with elevated BLLs, the benefits of secondary prevention, even when comprehensive follow-up care is provided, may be limited[37] for the following reasons.

- *Postponement of corrective action until after exposure means that children are forced to experience the harmful effects of lead.* Even after corrective actions are taken, reducing elevated BLLs is difficult because of the body burden of lead. Data from a recently conducted, multisite, randomized clinical trial indicate that chelation therapy, the recommended treatment for children with severely elevated BLLs ≥ 45 µg/dL, does not bring about improved neuropsychological outcome at 3-year follow-up among toddlers with preexisting BLLs 20 - 44 µg/dL.[38] This study confirms that chelation therapy does not reverse the neuropsychological effects of lead and underscores the need for preventing such effects.

- *Most blood lead screening is not performed when children are young enough to receive the full benefits of effective environmental interventions.* The timing of efforts to reduce exposure of children with elevated BLLs is critical. The BLLs of infants living in contaminated environments rise rapidly when these children are between the ages of 6 - 12 months[39] (the period at which crawling and mouthing behaviors are common). Often, by the time a child with an elevated BLL is identified through screening, he or she already has developed a large body burden of lead and is at increased risk for long-term health consequences. Environmental interventions (e.g., safe repair of deteriorated paint and reducing lead-contaminated dust in children's homes), that would effectively prevent BLL elevations in fetuses, infants, and young toddlers may not rapidly reduce the elevated BLL of a child who is no longer crawling and mouthing.

- *Correction of identified lead hazards in the child's home, an important aspect of responding to a child's elevated BLL, frequently may be delayed, inadequate, or nonexistent.* Deficiencies have been documented in the degree to which recommended interventions to reduce exposure, including remediating lead hazards and relocating families to lead-safe housing, actually are carried out (Pat McLaine RN, MPH, personal communication, CDC Region 1 Grantee Conference, November 1,2001).[40-42] Children with elevated BLLs are unlikely to reap maximum benefit from blood lead screening if appropriate medical follow-up is lacking[43] or if effective measures to control lead hazards are not subsequently employed. Successful control of lead hazards in properties where children were lead poisoned reduces the likelihood of future lead exposures and future cases of lead poisoning.[40]

Focus on Housing, the Primary Vector of Disease

Most children with BLLs ≥10 µg/dL have been exposed to dust and soil in and around older housing that has been contaminated with lead from deteriorated, lead-based paint. The nature and extent of the problem of deteriorated residential lead-based paint have been thoroughly investigated. Approximately 40% of all U.S. housing units (about 38 million homes) have some lead-based paint, and 25% of all U.S. housing units (about 24 million homes) have significant lead-based paint hazards.[44] Of units built before 1940, 68% have significant lead-based paint hazards, as do 43% of units built from 1940 to 1959. About 4.2 million units with some lead-based paint are occupied by families with children aged < 6 years. Young children in low-income families living in the 1.2 million housing units in the United States that have significant lead paint hazards as defined by HUD regulations are at highest risk for exposure to lead.[44]

Experience and recent developments in technology and national housing policy[†] make the implementation of housing-based primary prevention feasible on a larger scale. The following advancements have occurred within the last decade.

- Increased focus on low-income urban areas as disproportionately impacted by childhood lead exposure.

- Application of data mapping techniques that allows identification of neighborhoods and families whose children are at highest risk for lead exposure to ensure priority action.

- Expansion of knowledge about identification, control, and prevention of lead hazards, including recognition of the need to control, contain, and clean up lead dust during all activities that repair or disturb old paint.

- Expanded resources for lead hazard control.

- Requirements for notification regarding lead-based paint hazards at rental or sale of pre-1978 properties.

- Development of and wide accessibility to low cost tools for lead dust testing in order to identify hazards and provide clearance testing after completion of hazard control work.

---

† Enactment of federal legislation known as Title X in 1992 catalyzed a host of regulatory program, technologic, and policy changes at the federal, state, and local levels.

- Widespread availability of basic training in lead-safe work practices developed by HUD and the U.S. Environmental Protection Agency (EPA) and requirements to use lead-safe work practices in HUD-funded projects and federally assisted housing.

- Experience with implementation of state and local standards of care for lead safety.

- Establishment of the HUD requirement for Consolidated [housing] Plans to address lead safety.

Calls for expanding primary prevention efforts also have increased steadily.[45-52] In February 2000, the Federal Task Force on Environmental Health and Safety Risks to Children presented a 10-year plan for eliminating childhood lead poisoning, emphasizing that "the U.S. must immediately adopt a strategy to make housing lead-safe by eliminating lead-based paint hazards in the homes of children who are under the age of six years."[53]

Primary Prevention Program

The goal of targeting housing for primary prevention is to prevent adverse consequences of childhood lead exposure by removing the health hazards posed by lead-based paint and keeping homes "lead-safe." Primary prevention strategies must reflect geographic variation in the risk for lead exposure and must be designed to suit local circumstances, needs, and assets. Communities and homes at highest risk should receive the greatest attention and resources. CLPPPs in state and local health departments must identify these high-risk areas and provide the leadership needed to coordinate a successful effort to eliminate those risks before children experience elevated BLLs. Collaboration is essential among housing, community development, and code enforcement agencies; elected officials; federal agencies; property owners; and community-based organizations. The expansion of effective primary prevention initiatives will reduce the need for and increase the efficiency of delivery of appropriate secondary prevention services. In addition, because primary prevention efforts to create an adequate supply of lead-safe housing will be time consuming, CLPPPs should augment their systemic housing-based primary prevention programs with fast-track initiatives to identify families at highest risk who could benefit from immediate assessment and risk-reduction services.

Recommendations

The primary prevention capacities recommended in this section of the report comprise a framework for making housing lead-safe by 1) preventing future exposures and 2) protecting previously exposed children from further exposure. Some of the recommended measures will be most effective when carried out broadly (e.g., citywide training in lead-safe work practices and updating housing codes). Other activities should target areas where lead risk is highest (e.g., targeted code enforcement and community-based screening of housing at high risk for lead hazards). Other measures may be brought to the level of a specific property (e.g., when lead-associated hazard control efforts in the apartment of a child with an elevated BLL are extended to other apartments with similar lead hazards in the same building). In many cases, the activities in this report will be performed by organizations other than the local health department, including other public agencies, community groups, and the private sector including property owners and lead-abatement contractors. Public health agencies must provide leadership in educating others about lead safety and encouraging broad action to make housing "lead-safe." (See Appendix 1: Sample Roles and Responsibilities for Primary Prevention of Childhood Lead Poisoning.)

ACCLPP recommends the following eight elements as the foundation of a housing-based primary prevention program. Programs must be able to undertake the following activities to fully implement primary prevention.

1. Identify high-risk areas, populations, and activities associated with housing-based lead exposure by

    a.   Using surveillance, demographic, and housing data to identify high-risk geographic areas and to quantify progress in reducing childhood lead exposure and producing lead-safe housing units;

    b.   Using enhanced targeting strategies and information systems initially developed to improve lead screening for children to direct attention and expand resources to reduce lead hazards in high-risk housing, especially that occupied by at-risk families (i.e., low income with infants and/or expectant parents);

    c.   Identifying high-risk families who could benefit from immediate assessment and services to reduce their lead exposure risk. One efficient way of identifying and reaching such families is through existing programs that already have established relationships with communities or families at high risk for lead exposure (e.g.,Healthy Start [HS], Early Head Start [EHS], Special Supplemental Nutrition Program for Women, Infants and Children [WIC]), community health centers and managed Medicaid programs. Federal and state Medicaid agencies can consider incorporating lead exposure prevention services into newborn home-visiting requirements for high-risk populations and in high-risk areas.(See Appendix 2: Options for Targeting High-Risk Families with Young Children.);

d. Identifying individual families that may be living in dwellings with lead hazards. CLPPPs should use all tools at their disposal (e.g., elevated BLL case mapping, and environmental inspection and code violation reports) to identify families residing in dwellings with a high probability of having lead hazards. For example, families should receive priority attention if they live in a unit next to one in which a child with elevated BLLs has been identified; and

e. Giving high priority to identification and remediation of housing where multiple cases of childhood lead poisoning have been identified.

2. Use local data and expertise to expand resources and motivate action for primary prevention.

The systemic changes needed to implement primary prevention on a communitywide scale require new resources, agency commitment, political will, and community support. Securing such cooperation requires CLPPPs to present a persuasive rationale based on sound data. Health and housing agencies should use data to inform policy decisions and motivate action by

a. Presenting data about the problem to policymakers and community members and communicating the costs of inaction to the community and to affected families;

b. Highlighting risk disparities and identifying pockets of housing posing increased risk for lead poisoning;

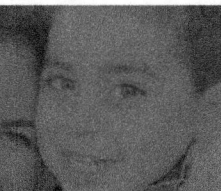

c.   Identifying a clear strategic plan and quantifying the resources necessary for success;

d.   Collaborating with housing agencies in the development of the lead hazard remediation component of the jurisdiction's Consolidated Plan for housing and community development investments;

e.   Encouraging effective and responsible media coverage;

f.   Using the federal Lead Hazard Disclosure law to increase property owners' motivation;

g.   Mobilizing community leadership among parents and others to develop neighborhood-based solutions, develop political will, and secure needed resources; and

h.   Identifying and reducing exposure to other sources of lead.

3. Develop strategies and ensure services for creating lead-safe housing.

Implementation of primary prevention requires that communities have an arsenal of different strategies for improving lead safety in various niches of the housing stock. Programs must ensure that a sufficient number of agencies and personnel are trained to provide lead-hazard evaluation and control services in their communities. Every effort should be made to integrate lead safety into other health and housing activities and to expand health department training and education to advance primary prevention. Examples of such integration follow.

a.   Identifying high-risk families for priority action to correct lead hazards. Such identification could be a routine part of all health department programs that identify and assist at-risk children and their families.

b.   Incorporating lead hazard screening, dust testing, and referral activities into home visits by health departments and other agency personnel. This would include providing training, tools, and protocols to screen for actual and potential lead exposures and linkage of screening activities with referral to agencies that can conduct environmental investigations and provide lead hazard control services, grants, or loans.

c. Implementing lead hazard control in priority properties.

d. Providing training in lead-safe work practices and dust sampling. This training could be offered to painters, renovators, code inspectors, weatherization contractors, realtors, property owners, and property managers.

e. Offering services (e.g., dust clearance testing and technical advice) to property owners as part of a public-private sector partnership.

f. Offering incentives to property owners for compliance with lead-safe housing treatments before children are poisoned.

g. Notifying tenants in adjacent units about possible lead hazards when a child is identified as lead poisoned in a multifamily building.

4. Develop and codify specifications for lead-safe housing treatments.

EPA regulations establish technical benchmarks for lead safety, and HUD guidelines describe how to perform various lead safety procedures. However, local jurisdictions must decide when and where to apply these tools to maximize lead safety, given local conditions.£ Specifically, local laws or regulations should require minimum lead-safe housing treatments for property repair and maintenance that ensure the differential treatment of various housing components on the basis of characteristics of the local housing stock, a property's risk, and the characteristics of the rental market.** For example, Maryland and Indiana require property owners to meet certain standards at property turnover and other key junctures. The result of codified housing standards is a clear understanding among all stakeholders of what is needed for a property to be considered lead-safe. Jurisdictions should ensure that such policies are developed in tandem with regulations designed to ensure adequate authority for government agencies to act if necessary. (See Recommendation 5 and Appendix 3: Developing and Codifying Specifications for Lead-Safe Housing Treatments.)

£HUD regulations controlling lead safety do not reach beyond federally assisted properties into the purely private (unassisted) housing stock, leaving decisions about regulating lead safety in this large portion of the affordable housing stock up to local jurisdictions

** Recent state laws have calibrated lead-safety measures to a property's risk, establishing tiered requirements for different circumstances, including 2002 laws enacted in Rhode Island and Maryland.

5. Strengthen regulatory infrastructure necessary to create lead-safe housing.

Laws and regulations should establish or clarify the legal authority of government agencies to ensure lead safety through enforcing housing codes, requiring lead-safe housing treatments by property owners (See Recommendation 4), and other necessary measures. (See Appendix 3: Developing and Codifying Specifications for Lead-Safe Housing Treatments.) These regulations should address

    a.   Lead-dust hazards and deteriorated paint as code violations;

    b.   Prohibition of unsafe work practices;

    c.   Postwork clearance dust-testing requirements; and

    d.   Enforcement through code violation citations, legally binding work orders, fines for noncompliance, direct administration, condemnation, and declaration of public nuisance.

The effectiveness of enforcement should be examined and changes made as needed to ensure protection of children.

6. Engage in collaborative plans and programs with housing and other appropriate agencies.

Match responsibilities and resources with needs to make and keep housing lead-safe. Essential elements in such collaborations are

    a.   Provision of leadership in fostering regular and substantive communication and collaboration among key public, community, and private sector entities. This includes developing partnerships with diverse groups, including parents of lead-poisoned children, community-based and advocacy organizations, retail outlets, lenders and insurers, property owners, home improvement and remodeling contractors, abatement contractors, and health-care providers;

b. Active participation in the provision of information on the location and extent of lead hazards and in development and execution of plans and activities to eliminate them, with particular emphasis on the HUD-required Consolidated Plan;[‡]

c. Pursuit of creative financing and subsidy strategies and assistance or incentives for voluntary lead-safety measures by owners of high-risk property; and

d. Consistent emphasis on lead-safe maintenance as a necessary element for lead safety in homes.

7. Evaluate and redesign existing CLPPP elements to achieve primary prevention goals while ensuring adequate secondary interventions.

Completing a shift to primary prevention requires a review of current programs so that priorities can be adjusted. Strengths of CLPPPs in identifying and working with families at highest risk could be used to prioritize individual families for services to ensure lead safety of their homes before exposure of their children. Some aspects of secondary prevention programs will be retained, others redirected, and some deferred. For example, CLPPPs should retain the capacity to ensure recommended blood lead screening and follow-up care for children with elevated BLLs. At the same time, the emphasis of health education activities could shift, for example, from providing general lead information to training contractors, property owners, and community members in lead-safe work practices. (See Appendix 4: Intersections of Primary and Secondary Prevention.)

---

‡ Jurisdictions receiving HUD Community Development Block Grant and HOME Housing Partnership funds are required to develop and update annually a Consolidated Plan that must address lead hazards. Specifically, as part of the needs assessment "the plan must estimate the number of housing units within the jurisdiction that are occupied by low-income families or moderate-income families that contain lead-based paint hazards" (24 CFR Part 91, Section 91.205 (e)) and the strategic plan "must outline the actions proposed or being taken to evaluate and reduce lead-based paint hazards, and describe how the lead-based paint hazard reduction will be integrated into housing policies and programs" (Ibid, Section 91.215 (g)). More generally, this section also provides "The consolidated plan must describe the jurisdiction's activities to enhance coordination between public and assisted housing providers and private and governmental health, mental health, and service agencies. With respect to the public entities involved, the plan must describe the means of cooperation and coordination among the State and any units of general local government in the metropolitan area in the implementation of its consolidated plan."

8. Evaluate primary prevention progress, and identify research opportunities.

a. CLPPPs should lead development and use of benchmarks and milestones for tracking the pace of primary prevention in their jurisdictions. They should ensure that local data guide decision making. Creative partnerships will be needed to evaluate primary prevention activity and progress. Systems for ongoing surveillance to capture children's BLLs across the full range of possible values and to track the presence and control of lead hazards in housing will be critical for measuring progress.

b. CLPPPs should identify and promote research opportunities as part of all ongoing primary prevention efforts. CLPPPs and their partners should simultaneously plan solid evaluations that will foster a better understanding of the effectiveness of their efforts. These evaluations will involve gathering baseline measures, systematically tracking program processes (i.e., interventions and costs) and measuring a variety of outcomes (in children, families, individual housing units, entire buildings and properties, neighborhoods, and communities). Additional research is needed to determine how to maintain safety for young children during application of primary prevention work, to refine lead safety interventions and standards, to measure the longevity and cost-effectiveness of preventive lead hazard control at various levels of intensity, to evaluate the efficacy of targeted educational efforts in reducing exposures, to evaluate the effectiveness of moving and maintaining young families in lead-safe housing, to determine the effectiveness of finance/subsidy strategies in creating lead-safe housing in targeted areas, to determine the effectiveness of applying lead hazard controls within neighborhoods to reduce cross-contamination of exterior hazards, and to evaluate community changes when regulatory mechanisms or guidelines are put into place. Federal agencies funding primary prevention efforts should consider the value of evaluation as part of any project proposal so that future commitments of resources can focus on successful approaches that cost-effectively achieve local and national goals.

Implementation of Primary Prevention

Specific examples of how these program elements are being implemented around the country are being documented through a CDC-funded project titled, *Building Blocks for Primary Prevention: Protecting Children from Lead-Based Paint Hazards*, which was initiated in October 2002. (See Appendix 5: Building Blocks for Primary Prevention: Protecting Children from Lead-Based Paint Hazards Project Synopsis.)

Appendix I. Sample Roles and Responsibilities for Primary Prevention of Childhood Lead Poisoning

Although the same general functions can be used as part of primary prevention efforts in different jurisdictions, the assignment of roles and responsibilities for carrying out those functions most likely will vary from place to place. ACCLPP recognizes that the institutional or legal environment, capacity of agencies and organizations, level of commitment, resources, competing priorities, and personalities of staff members can affect program plans and implementation. Thus, the following roles for the eight elements are provided as samples for consideration by local programs as they begin to collaborate with other entities to accomplish their program goals.

1. **Identify high-risk areas, populations, and activities associated with housing-based lead exposure.**
    a. Legislators: Ensure that state and local health and housing agencies have sufficient resources and legal authority to establish and maintain necessary health and housing data systems.

    b. Health and housing agencies: Collaborate on the analysis of locale-specific data to identify target areas.

    c. Child, health, and housing advocates: Advocate for policies and resources to support the establishment and maintenance of health, housing, and related data systems.

2. Use local data and expertise to expand resources and motivate action for primary prevention.
   a. Health and housing agencies:
      1) Disseminate information about housing that poses an increased risk for lead-associated health effects and the populations most likely to be affected to policymakers, media, and community stakeholders.

      2) Engage policymakers, property owners, insurers, contractors, and others in developing a strategic plan (including resource building) for the primary prevention of lead poisoning.

   b. Property owners, insurers, and contractors: Partner with government agencies to develop a strategic plan that establishes incentives and identifies resources for the primary prevention of lead poisoning.

   c. Child, health, and housing advocates: Develop local strategies for building community awareness of and value for lead safe housing, and political will to implement primary prevention.

3. Develop strategies and ensure services for creating lead-safe housing.
   a. Legislators:
      1) Evaluate and revise (as necessary) housing, health, and building codes to address lead safety.

      2) Fund and provide incentives for lead-related services (including lead hazard remediation, lead-safe work practices, and dust-clearance training for contractors, maintenance personnel, property owners, and others) and for emergency lead-safe housing for high-risk families.

      3) Fund the development of more safe and affordable housing.

   b. Health & housing agencies:
      1) Develop a strategy for improving existing housing to meet code and address lead safety.

2) Incorporate lead hazard screening, dust testing, referrals and minimum treatment standards into home visits.

3) Support training and provide technical assistance to property owners, contractors, and maintenance staff in lead-safe work practices and dust clearance testing.

4) Educate and provide services and/or referrals to high-risk families.

5) Build partnerships with property owners, insurers, and contractors to develop innovative, cost-effective, incentive-based strategies for making private sector housing lead-safe, especially distressed housing and housing in high-risk areas.

c. Property owners, insurers, and contractors: Partner with government agencies to develop cost-effective strategies for making private-sector housing lead-safe.

d. Child, health, and housing advocates:
   1) Advocate for enforcement and improvement of housing and building codes to address lead safety.

   2) Advocate for more safe and affordable housing.

   3) Identify and advocate for services for high-risk families.

4. Develop and codify specifications for lead-safe housing treatments.
   a. Legislators: Evaluate and revise (as necessary) existing housing and building codes to incorporate a lead-safe standard of care for housing that is consistent with research and evaluation findings.

   b. Health and housing agencies:
      1) Develop and implement systematic approaches to ongoing collection and analysis of dwelling-unit specific data, including lead-paint content, dust levels, and condition of components (e.g., doors, windows, and trim).

2) Collaborate with academic and research institutions to conduct systematic research and evaluation that can be used to support the development of a cost-effective, lead-safe standard of care for housing.

3) Disseminate findings to policymakers, media, and community stakeholders.

5. **Strengthen regulatory infrastructure to create lead-safe housing.**
   a. Legislators:
      1) Enact lead-safe housing standards.

      2) Fund enforcement activities.

      3) Monitor agency compliance.

   b. Health and housing agencies: Promote the updating or establishment of a regulatory structure for lead safety including housing code.

6. **Engage in collaborative plans and programs with housing and other appropriate agencies.**
   a. Legislators: Develop financing and subsidy strategies at the federal, state, and local levels.

   b. Health and housing agencies:
      1) Identify workload and resource needs to make high-risk housing lead-safe.

      2) Build public sector partnerships between agencies (e.g., the HUD-required Consolidated Plan).

      3) Build private sector partnerships (e.g., between property owners, insurers, and contractors).

   c. Property owners, insurers and contractors: Partner with government agencies to establish and implement plans for making and keeping private sector housing lead-safe, especially distressed housing.

    d.   Child, health & housing advocates:
        1) Educate constituents about lead safety.

        2) Build private sector partnerships.

        3) Advocate for adequate resources for lead
            poisoning prevention.

7. Evaluate and redesign existing CLPPP elements to achieve primary prevention goals while ensuring adequate secondary interventions.
    a.   Legislators: Provide adequate funding for lead poisoning prevention efforts.

    b.   Health and housing agencies:
        1) Assess existing programs: examine use of resources relative to primary and secondary prevention needs and evaluate the effectiveness of existing efforts.

        2) Engage stakeholders in developing strategies for increasing and redeploying resources to meet primary prevention needs.

8. Evaluate primary prevention progress, and identify research opportunities.
    a.   Legislators: Fund lead research and evaluation as priorities, as described.

    b.   Health and housing agencies:
        1) Develop evaluation plans.

        2) Design community-based research.

        3) Participate in programmatic research in collaboration with academic and community partners.

    c.   Property owners, insurers, contractors and others: Participate in planning and conduct of lead poisoning prevention research and evaluation studies.

d. Academic and research institutions:
   1) Collaborate with local health and housing agencies in conducting lead poisoning prevention research and programmatic evaluation.

   2) Disseminate research findings.

Appendix II. Options for Targeting High-Risk Families with Young Children

Until a sufficient stock of affordable, lead-safe housing is readily available, communities must take immediate steps to assist families who need lead hazard assessment and risk-reduction services. CLPPPs can use their expertise in the lead exposure patterns in their jurisdictions to implement efficient strategies to reach at-risk families. Once identified, such families should receive assessment of their children's lead exposure risk and services to help them prevent further exposure.

Identifying High-Risk Families

Several federal programs offer opportunities for efficient identification of and outreach to families with pregnant women and young children (e.g.,HS,EHS, and WIC). These programs recognize the influence of the prenatal and early childhood environment on child development, especially cognitive development, and the importance of early child development on later success in school and in life. Each program serves economically disadvantaged families who may be at increased risk for lead poisoning and can serve as a venue for initiating primary prevention activities. Because lead is a known developmental toxicant, ensuring that children are born into and grow up in a lead-safe environment should be integral to efforts to provide an environment that promotes optimal cognitive development. Provisions for assessment of lead-exposure risk and referral are not a formal part of these programs. Each program is described briefly below.

- *HS* supports community-based approaches to reducing infant mortality and improving the health and well being of women, infants, children, and their families. HS programs, which are administered by health departments or nonprofit organizations, serve 96 high-risk communities in 37 states. The federal Bureau of Maternal and Child Health in the Health Resources and Services Administration fund these programs. Although the focus of HS programs varies by community, collaborative opportunities between communities could be explored.

Appendix II

- *EHS* serves low-income families with infants, toddlers, and pregnant women.[54] Community programs supported by EHS provide early intervention services intended to enhance children's physical, social, emotional, and cognitive development. In addition, EHS aims to help parents improve their care-giving skills and meet their own goals, including economic independence. More than 600 EHS programs serve 45,000 low-income families with infants and toddlers. Features of EHS programs that are relevant to possible lead prevention activities include provision of assessments and services through home visits, when appropriate and a mandate to connect with other service providers at the local level to ensure that a comprehensive array of health, nutrition, and other services are available for families. EHS programs must begin with a community-needs assessment to guide design of the program and services offered. EHS prenatal education programs also must include information about other risks to optimal fetal development, including smoking and alcohol. Thus, adding an element of lead assessment, education, and intervention services in communities where lead exposure is prevalent among EHS families is consistent with other EHS efforts to ensure a healthy prenatal and postnatal environment.

- *WIC*, administered by the U.S. Department of Agriculture, serves low-income pregnant women and young children at risk for nutritional deficiencies. WIC provides supplemental nutritious foods, nutritional counseling, screening, and referral to other health and social services. WIC provides benefits to >7 million people each month, including 47% of all infants born in the United States.[55] Children served by WIC may be at high risk for exposures to lead. A Government Accounting Office analysis of Third National Health and Nutrition Examination Survey data found that 12% of children enrolled in the WIC program had elevated BLLs and that more than half of all children with such BLLs are members of families receiving WIC benefits.[56] In addition, a study in Wisconsin demonstrated that 60% of lead-poisoned children in Wisconsin receive WIC services.[57]

Strategies for Providing Assessment and Risk Reduction Services to At-Risk Families

The programs described in the preceding section offer efficient opportunities for reaching at-risk families. Following are possible approaches.

- *Assessment of lead exposure risk in the communities and populations served.* Through use of blood-lead screening, dust-lead screening, census data, and housing data, CLPPPs could identify HS, EHS, and WIC providers that serve communities or populations at high risk for lead poisoning.

- *Identification of individual clients who may be living in dwellings with lead hazards.* CLPPPs could undertake collaborative projects with HS, EHS, and WIC providers serving communities or populations at high risk for lead poisoning to use data linkage and other methods of identifying clients residing in dwellings with a high probability of lead hazards.

- *Addition of lead exposure risk assessment and referrals for lead inspections, lead hazard control, and relocation to lead-safe housing to program services.* CLPPPs could provide HS, EHS, and WIC programs serving populations at high-risk for lead poisoning with training, tools, and protocols to screen for potential lead exposures during client interviews and home visits. In addition, CLPPPs could refer families identified as having or being at high risk for exposure to lead hazards to agencies that can conduct environmental investigations and provide lead hazard control services, grants, or loans.

Appendix III. Developing and Codifying Specifications for Lead-Safe Housing Treatments

Housing can become lead-safe through the development and implementation of local strategies for making housing lead-safe and the use of local data to interpret how best to apply national standards for lead hazard control. States and localities are encouraged to develop lead-safe housing treatments that protect children while ensuring safe, affordable housing. Most jurisdictions have found that specifying required hazard treatments in law or regulation coupled with financial resources improves enforceability and community cooperation and increases understanding of the hazards prevalent in local housing stock.

Developing Local Policies for Lead-Safe Housing Treatments

In the early stage of developing local housing treatments, professionals face the challenge of recognizing that a minority of U.S. housing units (25%) contains lead-based paint hazards; therefore, a "one-size-fits-all" treatment plan is unlikely to be appropriate. However, the housing stock is a fluid entity; conditions change over time, so ongoing maintenance of the U.S. housing units in which lead-based paint has been identified (40% nationally)[44] is also of concern. Some states (e.g., Indiana and Rhode Island) have implemented tiered approaches that call for simple, baseline measures for all older housing, with more intensive interventions required in housing posing higher risk or in certain circumstances (e.g., in the home of a child identified as having elevated BLLs).[§] Policymakers can consider the following options for achieving lead-safe housing.

[§] For additional information about state laws, visit http://www.ncsl.org/programs/ESNR/cehdb.htm.

- *Baseline maintenance requirements for lead safety*-All owners of pre-1978 rental properties could be required to follow several baseline actions, including:

  O Avoiding unsafe work practices during maintenance, paint repair, and remodeling;
  O Performing routine visual inspections for paint deterioration;
  O Promptly and safely repairing deteriorated paint and its causes; and
  O Training property maintenance staff in lead-safe work practices.

  Unsafe Work Practices
  O Abrasive blasting
  O Power sanding without local exhaust ventilation
  O Open-flame burning
  O Dry sanding of large areas
  O Dry scraping of large areas

  Safe Work Practices: "work wet, work clean"
  O Minimization of dust generation
  O Wet scraping
  O Wet cleaning and HEPA vacuum
  O Dust testing following completion of work.

- *Additional requirements for properties posing higher risk*-Although baseline maintenance practices usually are sufficient to protect children in well-maintained properties, additional safeguards are needed in higher risk properties. In addition to identifying children with elevated BLLs, agencies could consider using housing events (e.g., vacancy, property sale, refinancing, and remodeling) as cues for owners of such properties to take additional safeguards, these include

  O Hire a certified lead-abatement contractor;
  O Control any identified lead-based-paint hazard;
  O Perform standard window treatments (usually abatement);
  O Plane doors to prevent binding;
  O Make floors smooth and cleanable; and
  O Pass dust clearance standards.

Related Regulatory Considerations

Recommendation 5 described basic authorities needed by health departments and other agencies to enforce lead safety requirements. Some jurisdictions may need additional authorities for full implementation, including the authority to

- Condition permits and licenses on compliance with lead safety standards;
- Inspect any rental unit and collect environmental samples;
- Prevent rent collection for properties in violation of codes;
- Require property owners to secure a lead inspection or risk assessment;
- Mandate that work be performed by a certified lead-abatement contractor;
- Place liens on properties to recover costs incurred for repairs by city-sponsored crews;
- Place properties in receivership;
- Declare a property with lead hazards a public nuisance; and
- Notify families in multifamily buildings of the possibility of lead paint hazards.

Appendix III

Appendix IV. Intersections of Primary and Secondary Prevention

Many tools needed for successful case management[3] also are needed for primary prevention. These include a description of the problem; targeting of children at highest risk for priority action (e.g., blood lead screening and lead hazard reduction); delineation of effective and feasible housing treatments; and broad collaboration to secure both public and private resources to promptly eliminate lead-based paint hazards. Specific examples of the application of expertise in secondary prevention toward primary prevention are presented below.

• *Lead hazard control in the homes of children with elevated BLLs.* Lead hazard control work should, at a minimum, be performed by persons knowledgeable about lead-safe work practices and be followed by clearance testing to confirm that lead dust hazards are not left behind at completion of the work.[3, 53, 58] Such action not only protects the children already identified as having elevated BLLs, but also accomplishes primary prevention for younger siblings or for the next family that occupies a lead-safe property. The challenge is how to bring about systemic change that will make these activities routine rather than rare.

• *Targeting.* Ongoing efforts to intensify screening among children at highest risk for lead exposure will provide a crucial point of intersection for secondary and primary prevention efforts.[59,60] The housing in areas selected for intensified blood-lead screening campaigns should be the target of screening to identify housing units that could be hazardous to present or future occupants. Homes of children <1 year of age also can be targeted using birth certificate data. Results from such screening would lay the foundation for remediation of identified lead-based paint hazards. Families targeted for blood lead screening could receive priority action to achieve lead safety in their homes before their children become exposed.

- *Surveillance.* CLPPPs have developed data systems that allow them to link information from disparate sources. These systems can be the foundation for initiatives that allow linking and exchange of critical information about populations, housing stock, and risk factors, including the addresses of homes where children have been poisoned or where lead hazards have been documented. Surveillance of housing stock through visual exterior assessments, followed by dust testing if deteriorated paint is observed is important to maintaining a stock of lead-safe housing. The condition of housing changes over time. For example, lead hazard reduction, whether triggered by identification of a lead-poisoned child and subsequent environmental investigation or through screening of housing and code enforcement, takes place at a point in time. Conditions in a home may deteriorate after remediation, and a home that was once "lead-safe" can develop new lead hazards over time. Housing registries and integrated surveillance systems enable communities to track housing condition, thereby supporting primary prevention.

- *Technology transfer from secondary to primary prevention.* Various stakeholders in the secondary prevention of childhood lead exposure have contributed to the development of a vast body of information, knowledge, and experience about lead safety and ways to establish, improve, and maintain it. All of this accumulated wisdom must be used to address primary prevention. For example, housing in which lead hazards have been identified and reduced could be the focal point of efforts to expand training in routine maintenance and repair. Health departments can sponsor training in lead dust sampling and help contractors gain certification. CLPPP staff can educate local and state elected officials and help revise housing codes to incorporate lead safety.

Appendix V. Building Blocks for Primary Prevention: Protecting Children from Lead-Based Paint Hazards Project Synopsis

Building Blocks for Primary Prevention: Protecting Children from Lead-Based Paint Hazards is a wide-ranging collection of promising strategies. The primary audience is state and local health departments who will be able to implement strategies by coordinating or encouraging action by other government agencies, community-based organizations, and the private sector. The strategies target persons living in high-risk properties and neighborhoods; screening housing at increased risk for lead hazards; strengthening code enforcement; using enforcement in tandem with subsidies; increasing rental property owners' motivation; leveraging the federal disclosure law; using data for full effect; engaging the media; increasing consumer demand; building political will; improving accountability; creating new partnerships; building capacity for lead safety services; integrating lead-safety into existing systems; expanding subsidies and dedicated resources; developing innovative financing mechanisms; and linking secondary and primary prevention.

In contrast with case studies that analyze one program in-depth, this project will summarize individual strategies. Wherever possible, each summary, or building block, will be illustrated using an example, with contact information provided for the program(s) featured. For consideration, strategies must embody sensitivity to housing affordability; principles of public health; potential for broad-scale impact; feasibility; and promise of success in reducing lead and other environmental health hazards in housing that poses an increased risk.

The Alliance for Healthy Homes is developing summaries of an estimated 50-100 Building Blocks under contract with CDC's Lead Poisoning Prevention Branch, Emergency and Environmental Health Services, National Center for Environmental Health. For more information, visit www.afhh.org.

Appendix VI. Resources

National Lead Information Center
Funded by the U.S. Environmental Protection Agency;
U.S. Department of Health and Human Services;
and the U.S. Department of Housing and Urban Development
Phone: 800-424-LEAD (800-424-5323)
Fax: 585-232-3111
Website: http://www.epa.gov/lead/nlic
E-mail address: See website
Address:　　National Lead Information Center
　　　　　　　　424 South Clinton Avenue
　　　　　　　　Rochester, NY 14620

U.S. Consumer Product Safety Commission
Phone:　800-638-2772 or 800-638-8270
　　　　　　(for the hearing and speech impaired)
Fax: 301-504-0124 and 301-504-0025
Website: http://www.cpsc.gov
E-mail address: info@cpsc.gov
Address:　　U.S. Consumer Product Safety Commission
　　　　　　　　Washington, DC 20207-0001

U.S. Department of Health and Human Services Public Health Service
Agency for Toxic Substances and Disease Registry (ATSDR)
Phone:　888-42-ATSDR (888-422-8737)
Fax: 404-498-0093
Website: http://www.atsdr.cdc.gov
E-mail address: ATSDRIC@cdc.gov
Address:　　ATSDR
　　　　　　　　1600 Clifton Road, N.E.
　　　　　　　　Atlanta, GA 30333

Appendix VI

U.S. Department of Health and Human Services Public Health Service
Centers for Disease Control and Prevention
National Center for Environmental Health
Lead Poisoning Prevention Branch
Phone: 770-488-3300
Fax: 770-488-3635
Website: http://www.cdc.gov.nceh/lead
E-mail address: leadinfo@cdc.gov
Address: 4770 Buford Highway MS F-40
                Atlanta, GA 30341

U.S. Department of Health and Human Services Public Health Service
Centers for Disease Control and Prevention
National Institute for Occupational Safety and Health
Phone: 800-35-NIOSH (800-356-4674)
Fax: 513-533-8573 or 888.232.3299
Website: http://www.cdc.gov/niosh
E-mail address: eidtechinfo@cdc.gov
Address: 4676 Columbia Parkway
                Cincinnati, OH 45226

U.S. Department of Health and Human Services Public Health Service
National Institutes of Health
National Library of Medicine
Toxicology and Environmental Health Information
Phone: 888-FINDNLM (888-346-3656)
Fax: 301-480-3537
Website: http://sis.nlm.nih.gov
E-mail address: tehip@teh.nlm.nih.gov
Address: Specialized Information Services NLM/NIH
                2 Democracy Plaza, Suite 510
                6707 Democracy Boulevard, MSC 5467
                Bethesda, MD 20892-5467

U.S. Department of Housing and Urban Development
Office of Healthy Homes and Lead Hazard Control
Phone: 202-755-1785
Fax: 202-755-1000
Website: http://www.hud.gov/offices/lead
E-mail address: lead_regulations@hud.gov
Address: 451 7th Street, SW
                Room P3206
                Washington, DC 20410

U.S. Department of Labor
Occupational Safety and Health Administration
Phone: 800-321-OSHA (800-321-6742) or 877-889-5627 (for the hearing and speech impaired)
Fax: none
Website: http://www.osha.gov
E-mail address: See website
Address: U.S. Department of Labor Occupational
            Safety and Health Administration
            200 Constitution Avenue, NW
            Washington, DC 20210

U.S. Environmental Protection Agency
Office of Pollution Prevention and Toxics
Phone: 202-566-0500
Fax: 202-566-0469
Website: http://www.epa.gov/lead/
E-mail address: See website
Address: US EPA/Lead
            Office of Pollution Prevention and Toxics
            1200 Pennsylvania Avenue, NW
            Mail Code 7404T
            Washington, DC 20460

PRIVATE ORGANIZATIONS

Alliance for Healthy Homes (Formerly the Alliance to End Childhood Lead Poisoning)
Phone: 202-543-1147
Fax: 202-543-4466
Website: http://www.afhh.org
E-mail address: afhh@afhh.org
Address: 227 Massachusetts Avenue, NE
            Suite 200
            Washington, DC 20002

American Public Health Association
Phone: 202-777-APHA (202-777-2742)
Fax: 202-777-2534
Website: http://www.apha.org
E-mail address: comments@apha.org
Address: 800 I Street, NW
            Washington, DC 20001-3710

The National Center for Healthy Housing
Phone: 410-992-0712
Fax: 410-715-2310
Website: http://www.centerforhealthyhousing.org
E-mail address: nchh@enterprisefoundation.org
Address: 10227 Wincopin Circle, Suite 100
Columbia, MD 21044-3400

National Low Income Housing Coalition
Phone: 202-662-1530
Fax: 202-393-1973
Website: http://www.nlihc.org
E-mail address: info@nlihc.org
Address: 1012 14th Street NW, Suite 610
Washington, DC 20005

National Conference of State Legislatures
Phone: 303-364-7700
Fax: 303-364-7800
Website: www.ncsl.org
E-mail: info@nscl.org
Address: 7700 East First Place
Denver, CO 80230

References

[1] U.S. Department of Health and Human Services. Healthy People 2010: Understanding and Improving Health. Washington, DC: U.S. Department of Health and Human Services, Office of Disease Prevention and Health Promotion; 2000. Available at: URL: http://www.healthypeople.gov/Document/HTML/Volume1/08Environmental.htm#_Toc490564711: Accessed 11/3/03

[2] CDC. Second National Report on Human Exposure to Environmental Chemicals. Atlanta: U.S. Department of Health and Human Services, CDC; 2003 (Publication no. 02-0716). Available at: URL: http://www.cdc.gov/exposurereport. Accessed 11/3/03

[3] CDC. Managing elevated blood lead levels among young children: Recommendations from the Advisory Committee on Childhood Lead Poisoning Prevention. Atlanta: U.S. Department of Health and Human Services, CDC; 2002. Available at: URL: http://www.cdc.gov/nceh/lead/CaseManagement/caseManage_main.htm. Accessed 11/03/03.

[4] CDC. Preventing lead poisoning in young children. Atlanta: U.S. Department of Health and Human Services, CDC; 1991.

[5] CDC. Update: blood lead levels-United States, 1991-1994. MMWR Morb Mortal Wkly Rep 1997;46:141 - 6 [published erratum MMWR Morb Mortal Wkly Rep 1997;46:607].

[6] Brody DJ, Pirkle JL, Kramer RA, et al. Blood lead levels in the US population: Phase 1 of the Third National Health and Nutrition Examination Survey (NHANES III, 1988 to 1991). JAMA 1994;272:277 - 83.

[7] Pirkle JL, Brody DJ, Gunter EW, et al. The decline in blood lead levels in the United States: The National Health and Nutrition Examination Surveys (NHANES). JAMA 1994:272:284 - 91.

[8] Grosse SD, Matte TD, Schwartz J, Jackson RJ. Economic gains resulting from the reduction in children's exposure to lead in the United States. Environ Health Perspect 2002;110:563 - 9.

[9] Flegal AR, Smith DR. Lead levels in preindustrial humans [letter]. N Engl J Med 1992;326:1293 - 4.

[10] Canfield RL, Henderson CR Jr, Cory-Slechta DA, Cox C, Jusko TA, Lanphear BP. Intellectual impairment in children with blood lead concentrations below 10 g per deciliter. N Engl J Med 2003;348:1517 - 26.

[11] Bellinger DC, Needleman HL. Intellectual impairment and blood lead levels [letter]. N Engl J Med 2003;349:500 - 2.

[12] Selevan SG, Rice DC, Hogan KA, Euling SY, Pfahles-Hutchens A, Bethel J. Blood lead concentration and delayed puberty in girls. N Engl J Med 2003;348:1527 - 36.

[13] Wu T, Buck GM, Mendola P. Blood lead levels and sexual maturation in U.S. girls: the Third National Health and Nutrition Examination Survey, 1988 - 1994. Environ Health Perspect 2003;111:737 - 41.

[14]Pirkle JL, Kaufmann RB, Brody DJ, Hickman T, Gunter EW, Paschal DC. Exposure of the U.S. population to lead, 1991 - 1994. Environ Health Perspect 1998;106:745 - 50.

[15]Gellert GA, Wagner GA, Maxwell RM, Moore D, Foster L. Lead poisoning among low-income children in Orange County, California. A need for regionally differentiated policy. JAMA 1993;270:69 - 71.

[16]Parry C, Eaton J. Kohl: a lead-hazardous eye makeup from the Third World to the First World. Environ Health Perspect 1991;94:121 - 3.

[17]Matte TD, Proops D, Palazuelos E, Graef J, Hernandez Avila M. Acute high-dose lead exposure from beverage contaminated by traditional Mexican pottery. Lancet 1994;344:1064 - 65.

[18]Norman EH, Hertz-Picciotto I, Salmen D, Ward T. Childhood lead poisoning and vinyl miniblind exposure. Arch Pediatr Adolesc Med 1997:151:1033 - 37.

[19]Baker EL, Folland DS, Taylor TA, et al. Lead poisoning in children of lead workers: home contamination with industrial dust. N Engl J Med 1977;296:260 - 1.

[20]Roscoe RJ, Gittleman JL, Deddens JA, Petersen MR, Halperin WE. Blood lead levels among children of lead-exposed workers. A meta-analysis. Am J Ind Med 1999;36:475 - 81.

[21]Roberts TM, Hutchinson TC, Paciga J, Chattopadhyay A, Jervis RE, Van Loon J. Lead contamination around secondary smelters: estimation of dispersal and accumulation by humans. Science 1974;186:1120 - 22.

[22]Roels HA, Buchet JP, Lauwerys RR, et al. Exposure to lead by the oral and the pulmonary routes of children living in the vicinity of a primary lead smelter. Environ Res 1980;22:81 - 94.

[23]Kosatsky T, Boivin MC. Blood lead levels in children living near abandoned metal-recovery plants. Can J Public Health 1994;85:158 - 62.

[24]Murgueytio AM, Evans RG, Sterling DA, Clardy SA, Shadel BN, Clements BW. Relationship between lead mining and blood lead levels in children. Arch Environ Health 1998;53:414 - 23.

[25]Hilts SR. Effect of smelter emission reductions on children's blood lead levels. Sci Total Environ 2003;303:51 - 8.

[26]Lanphear BP, Burgoon DA, Rust SW, Eberly S, Galke W. Environmental exposures to lead and urban children's blood lead levels. Environ Res 1998;76:120 - 30.

[27]Amitai Y, Brown MJ, Graef JW, Cosgrove E. Residential deleading: effects on the blood lead levels of lead-poisoned children. Pediatrics 1991;88:893 - 7.

[28]Reissman DB, Matte TD, Gurnitz KL, Kaufmann RB, Leighton J. Is home renovation or repair a risk factor for exposure to lead among children residing in New York City? J Urban Health 2002;79:502 - 11.

[29]Lanphear BP, Howard C, Eberly S, et al. Primary prevention of childhood lead exposure: a randomized trial of dust control. Pediatrics 1999;103:772 - 7.

[30]Institute of Medicine (U.S.). Committee for the Study of the Future of Public Health. The Future of Public Health. Washington, DC: National Academy Press; 1988.

[31]CDC. Strategic Plan for the Elimination of Childhood Lead Poisoning. Atlanta: US Department of Health and Human Services, CDC; 1991.

[32]CDC. Program Announcement 03007. Childhood Lead Poisoning Prevention Programs (CLPPP) Notice of Availability of Funds, January 2003. Available at: URL: http://www.cdc.gov/od/pgo/funding/03007.htm. Accessed 11/03/03.

[33]National Research Council. Measuring Lead Exposure in Infants, Children, and Other Sensitive Populations. Washington, DC: National Academy Press; 1993.

[34]Meyer P, Pivetz T, Dignam T, Homa D, Schoonover J, Brody D. Surveillance for elevated blood lead levels among children-United States, 1997 - 2000. MMWR Morb Mortal Wkly Rep 2003;52(SS-10)1 - 20. Available at: URL: http://www.cdc.gov/mmwr/preview/mmwrhtml/ss5210a1.htm#tab1. Accessed 11/03/03.

[35]Liu X, Dietrich KN, Radcliffe J, Ragan B, Rhoads GG, Rogan WJ. Do children with falling blood lead levels have improved cognition? Pediatrics 2002;110:787 - 91.

[36]Tong S, Baghurst PA, Sawyer MG, Burns J, McMichael AJ. Declining blood lead levels and changes in cognitive function during childhood: the Port Pirie Cohort Study. JAMA 1998;280:1915 - 9.

[37]Leighton J, Klitzman S, Sedlar S, Matte T, Cohen NL. The effect of lead-based paint hazard remediation on blood lead levels of lead poisoned children in New York City. Environ Res 2003;92:182 - 90.

[38]Rogan WJ, Dietrich KN, Ware JH, et al. The effect of chelation therapy with succimer on neuropsychological development in children exposed to lead. N Engl J Med 2001;344:1421 - 6.

[39]Tong S, Baghurst P, McMichael A, Sawyer M, Mudge J. Lifetime exposure to environmental lead and children's intelligence at 11 - 13 years: the Port Pirie cohort study. BMJ 1996;312:1569 - 75. [erratum BMJ 1996;313:198].

[40]Brown MJ, Gardner J, Sargent JD, Swartz K, Hu H, Timperi R. The effectiveness of housing policies in reducing children's lead exposure. Am J Public Health 2001;91:621 - 4.

[41]Perez L. An epidemic of neglect: lead poisoning prevention often comes too little, too late. Syracuse, NY: The Herald-American, 2001 (July 22): A1.

[42]Wenland-Bowyer W, Lam T, Christensen M. Worst Michigan neighborhoods: lead-poisoned blocks pinpointed. Detroit, MI: The Detroit Free Press, 2003 (July 29): 1A, 5A.

[43]Markowitz M, Rosen JF, Clemente I. Clinician follow-up of children screened for lead poisoning. Am J Public Health 1999;89:1088 - 90.

[44]Jacobs DE, Friedman W, Clickner RP, et al. The prevalence of lead-based paint hazards in U.S. Housing. Environ Health Perspect 2002;110:599 - 606. Available at: http://www.hud.gov/offices/lead/techstudies/HUD_NSLAH_Vol1.pdf. Accessed 11/03/03.

[45]Binder S, Matte T. Childhood lead poisoning: the impact of prevention. JAMA 1993;269:1679 - 81.

[46]Lanphear BP. The paradox of lead poisoning prevention. Science 1998;282:51.

[47]Needleman HL. Childhood lead poisoning: the promise and abandonment of primary prevention. Am J Public Health 1998;88:1871 - 77.

[48]Ryan D, Levy B, Pollack S, Walker B Jr. Protecting children from lead poisoning and building healthy communities. Am J Public Health 1999;89:822 - 4.

[49]Campbell C, Osterhoudt KC. Prevention of childhood lead poisoning. Curr Opin Pediatr 2000;12:428 - 37.

[50]Satcher DS. The Surgeon General on the continuing tragedy of childhood lead poisoning. Public Health Rep 2000;115:579 - 80.

[51]Rosen J, Mushak P. Primary prevention of childhood lead poisoning-the only solution. N Engl J Med 2001;344:1470 - 1.

[52]Lanphear BP, Dietrich KN, Berger O. Prevention of lead toxicity in US children. Ambul Pediatr 2003;3:27 - 36.

[53]President's Task Force on Environmental Health. Risks and Safety Risks to Children Eliminating Childhood Lead Poisoning. A Federal Strategy Targeting Lead Paint Hazards. Washington, DC; February 2000.

[54]U.S. Department of Health and Human Services, Administration for Children & Families, Health Start Bureau. "Early Health Start," last modified 06/07/02. Available at: URL: http://www.acf.dhhs.gov/programs/hsb/programs/ehs/ehs.htm. Accessed 11/03/03.

[55]U.S. Department of Agriculture, WIC: The Special Supplemental Nutrition Program for Women, Infants, and Children. Nutrition Program Facts, Food and Nutrition Service. Wash. DC: USDA; 2002 Available at: URL: http://www.fns.usda.gov/wic/wic-fact-sheet.pdf. Accessed 11/03/03.

[56]U.S. General Accounting Office. Lead Poisoning: Federal Health Care Programs are Not Effectively Reaching at Risk Children. Washington, DC: US General Accounting Office, 1998; GAO publication no. GAO/HEHS-98-169R.

[57]LaFlash S, Joosse-Coons M, Havlena J, Anderson HA. Wisconsin children at risk for lead poisoning. Wis Med J 2002;99:18 - 22.

[58]U.S. Department of Housing and Urban Development. Guidelines for the Evaluation and Control of Lead-Based Paint Hazards in Housing. Washington, DC: U.S. HUD 1539-LBP; 1995.

[59]CDC. Recommendations for blood lead screening of young children enrolled in Medicaid: targeting a group at high risk. Advisory Committee on Childhood Lead Poisoning Prevention (ACCLPP). MMWR Morb Mortal Wkly Rep 2000;49(RR-14).

[60]CDC. Screening Young Children for Lead Poisoning: Guidance for State and Local Public Health Officials. Atlanta: U.S. Department of Health and Human Services, CDC;